THE LONG GOODBYE

Lewy Body Dementia – Alzheimer's First Cousin

BARBARA J. SECKLIN

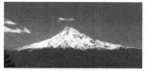

Shara † Basha
Publishing

ISBN: 1511441372
ISBN-13: 978-1511441377

For all of my children.
They make me proud to be
their mother.

CONTENTS

DUST

In time to come don't look for me
In sacred space, in hallowed halls
In stone-carved, cold unchanging ground -
I won't be found.

In crypted stately columned room
In crystal silent drift of dreams
In holy, candle-scented air -
I won't be there.

My mortal dust has taken flight
To rise and kiss the sun-lit sky
To sift through shadowed, dancing leaves
And fall on roses with the rain
To shout and whisper with the wind
In deserts, lakes, and mountain's stair -
Oh, I'll be there!

And when in spring the robin wings -
There - my heart sings.

Lewy body dementias (LBD) affect an estimated 1.4 million individuals and their families in the United States, yet few individuals and medical professionals are aware of the symptoms, diagnostic criteria, or even that LBD exists. An increasing number of general practitioners, neurologists and other medical professionals are beginning to learn to recognize and differentiate the symptoms of LBD – but it remains the most misdiagnosed dementia – from other diseases.

More research is needed. With further research, LBD may ultimately be treated and prevented through early detection and neuroprotective interventions. Currently, there is no specific test to diagnose LBD.

Lewy Body Dementia Association, Inc.

10 Things You Should Know about LBD

CHAPTER 1

"I can't run. I'm dizzy."

My husband stood just inside our front door. He had gone out of the house not even ten minutes earlier that morning, heading out onto the back road behind our property for his daily four and a half mile run. Now, he asked for another cup of coffee, crossed over to the living room sofa, and flipped on the television set. I didn't know it then, but the couch and the TV set were to be the most outstanding features throughout the remainder of his life.

I remember questioning him that morning, idly discussing the possibility that he was coming down with a cold. How else do you address a statement so insignificant and unspecific as, "I'm dizzy."? You chalk it up to inner ear pressure or possibly something he ate. "It'll be fine," you say. "You'll run tomorrow."

But the next morning was the same. And the following day. He certainly wasn't ill. Nothing hurt. Nothing really specific, except for that one ridiculous symptom. He was dizzy. And I have to reiterate these words – Nothing really specific. This was true throughout his illness, and research seems to reflect it: Symptoms of Lewy Body Dementia? Nothing really specific. What results are shown with testing? Nothing really specific.

"I'm dizzy, I can't run."

And just that simply began a nine-year odyssey – a journey –not of discovery and enlightenment, but one of confusion and frustration. We never got any answers. No one was ever able to give me satisfactory reasons to explain exactly what was wrong. And this 'not knowing', this uncertain feeling seemed to isolate us in a limbo of being unable to DO anything. The natural order of things is:

A. Find out what's wrong.

B. Fix it. And...

C. Get on with your life.

Simple, right? That's what everyone does. But, we just couldn't.

The very *non*-importance of the beginning of it has made me a little unsure of exactly what day, what month it started. While I'm vague on when exactly it started, the circumstances, however, are carved deep into my mind because that day marked the start of major changes. The division between then and now. Between two totally different lifestyles.

From active, busy-every-day lives, to a completely sedentary existence. From being social folks with a large circle of interesting friends and acquaintances – to living as sequestered hermits. From being happy travelers, campers and explorers – to our new identity of being stay at home stick-in-the-muds.

Comparing who we were to who we

became doesn't add to the scientific knowledge of this disease, I know, but it seems to be a large part of how so many people must deal with it. Of course, I can only speak for myself, but at the conclusion I can look back and say that not only were *we* changed, but so was our entire family, our health, our future, our friends, our home; everything.

CHAPTER 2

Perhaps Lewy Body Dementia (LBD) strikes in a different pattern for every family it happens to, affecting individuals differently, with different ways of dealing with it. I don't know. When it happened to us, it arrived quietly, with just that one persistent symptom: dizziness. And it went on to take over our lives with a steady, grinding devastation.

What is Lewy Body Dementia? According to the Lewy Body Dementia Association website: "LBD is not a rare disease. It affects an estimated 1.4 million individuals and their families in the United States. Because LBD symptoms can closely resemble other more commonly known diseases like Alzheimer's and Parkinson's, it is currently widely underdiagnosed. Many doctors and other medical professionals still are not familiar with LBD." The LBD Association website offers abundant information.

For further research, here is their link:

http://www.lbda.org/category/3437/what-is-lbd.htm

* * *

My husband was at that time, in his early seventies; I was three years older. We lived in a valley in central Arizona on top of a hill, near a small town, surrounded by magnificent scenery. Comfortably retired, we indulged ourselves in travel, sightseeing, and long camping trips. We also ventured out on occasional cross-country trips to visit our widely scattered family.

Much of our activities and social life

centered around the fact that we belonged to a local gem and mineral club. My husband was, at the time, vice-president and membership chairman; I was on the board of directors. We participated in all the various functions the club was involved in.

Together, we led field trips, put on fireside talks at the state park, taught wire-wrapping classes, gave learning talks at the local library, attended all meetings and club-related functions. As club representatives, we participated in other annual regional festivities: river days, birding and nature festivals, and mining-related occasions. We helped organize and put on the club's annual gem show, an event that was very well known throughout the southwest.

When not involved in club activities, we hiked mountain trails, explored and sought out new camping spots, spent extended weekends at the state's beautiful lakes and reservoirs, visited friends, went sight-seeing. We were always busy.

So, obviously, we had stayed active. We ran, walked, biked, and swam. Of course our diet was a healthy one. We watched what we ate. We kept reasonable hours. We had no questionable drug or drinking habits.

We had a pleasant, fulfilling social life.

Oh my goodness, weren't we wonderful, model senior citizens?

Are you getting the picture here? It seems apparent that Lewy Body Dementia has nothing to do with one's physical or mental or emotional health. It just happens. Unbidden, undeserved, it just happens. Perhaps in the future, the researchers will be able to pinpoint a cause, but as of this writing, the cause is unknown.

Back to my narrative.

Later that day − the day he didn't run.

At lunchtime, he pushed his plate aside, telling me that *eating* made the dizziness worse.

The following several days shaped a new pattern for him. He would get up early, leave the house to make an attempt at running, then return after five or ten minutes and head right back to the couch. Walking was tried. Biking too. Those also made him dizzy. The dizziness became a new, unwanted dweller in our home. It seldom left, and there were a multitude of things that made it worse.

Through trial and error, we found that

he *could* eat, but only after around seven P.M. And how truly odd is that? So, that became our new dinnertime. And since he was hungry again later, he developed a habit of midnight snacking. During this week…two weeks?…activity of any kind produced an increase in the strange dizziness. Driving quickly became out of the question too. Imagine the concern over the chances of causing an accident. Or injuring someone.

CHAPTER 3

Let's talk for a moment about diagnosis. As it turned out for us, that was a pretty elusive thing to find. Being fairly reasonable people, we made an appointment with his family doctor. More than one appointment. Presenting yourself at the doctor's office with such a vague, indefinite set of symptoms? Challenging, to say the least, for everyone concerned.   People   are   only human, after all. There was a strong tendency for many people to pause, look at him and say, "That's it? That's all? You're *dizzy*?"

And so the testing started. Blood tests, X-rays, scans, all the ins and outs of the local hospital and other local facilities. Over the entire span of years, I've lost track of the number of tests that were done. The number of prescriptions he tried. The number of appointments that we dutifully trudged off to keep, waited for results, and again were informed that the results were negative or inconclusive. "Nothing specific."

And the search began to spread. Other doctors were sought out. He saw some specialists. When all he could explain to them was that he had the one symptom of being dizzy, which was made worse by activity and by eating earlier than seven in the evening…well, let's just say that the reactions were often very interesting. Maybe ten years ago Lewy Body Dementia hadn't been heard of. Or was only known within the precincts of research.

Back to the question of diagnosis. Elusive? Let me change that. Invisible is more like it. We struggled through the entire eight to ten years without any definitive idea of what was wrong. The possibilities, however, were numerous. Depression. Lyme disease. Hypothyroid condition. Low testosterone. Mini-strokes. Inner ear problems. Blocked carotid artery. Brain tumor. Parkinson's disease. It could be the early onset of *anything*. The list seemed endless, and so did the medications. To be very precise, nothing worked, nothing alleviated the dizziness.

In the interest of total information disclosure, I have to include here some mention of my husband's particular nature.

Like all very intelligent people, he was a multi-faceted individual. He did an enormous amount of reading and information gathering. Unfortunately, he trusted his own opinions above those of others, even that of experts and professionals.

This led to a certain type of arrogance that had him self-diagnosing and self-medicating. To seeking out advice, supplements, and treatments on the internet. To deciding that some doctor-suggested test was unnecessary. To stop taking pills, or to cut them in half. He outright refused an MRI of his head.

It seems odd to find this in someone who has spent a lifetime interested in the pursuit of health, exercise, a proper diet, etc. It was frustrating to the doctors, to me, and to our whole family. Several family members still hold the opinion that *if only* he'd done this or that, the outcome would have been different.

He also had the misfortune to suffer with an intermittent OCD condition. This was contained and managed fairly well his entire life, so that it was not overwhelming. I think I can safely say that it was more of a problem and burden for him than it was for me or for the rest of the family. However, that too was soon to change.

CHAPTER 4

As the months passed, he started to develop a nagging concern over various things. He could no longer tolerate newspapers or magazines in the house. He would read an article, and then worry that he'd "forget" it, so he'd have to read it again, or better yet, make a few copies of it so that the information wouldn't get "lost". I began finding him in the living room at two or three in the morning, re-reading something in order to "remember" it. So eventually, it became easier to simply ban those publications from the house.

He started to become anxious over my whereabouts, not wanting me to be gone from home for any extended length of time. Even if I was occupied with some chore in another room, he'd call out, asking me to bring it to where he was and do it there. And he became less willing to have any guests come to the house, saying he "just didn't really feel up to it."

I'm not sure if you'd call them actual

symptoms of the developing LBD, or if what I was seeing was just an exacerbation of previously existing conditions, or did one cause the other; I'll leave that to the experts. But his OCD returned and worsened. His concerns quickly became worries and later turned into full-blown, time-consuming anxieties. There now was no limit to his range of things to be anxious about.

He decided that the air-conditioning unit was sure to fail, and then he would get too hot. His temperature perception had now gone awry. Another LBD symptom? (At that time, we didn't know that it was.) His "feeling too hot" began to control our life; he could not go any place where they might keep it too hot. No cars either; even if they had AC. What if an accident occurred and we had to walk in the heat of the sun?

Then there came another thing to add to dizzy and too hot. Sensitive eyes. Too much light was intolerable, so we had to keep the blinds closed. Not halfway either. Completely shut. Anywhere we went – to a medical appointment, to our daughter's home, to his dentist – he would request that they lower the temperature and shut the curtains or blinds. And by the way, could anyone locate a fan for him?

He was sure that the septic system was about to disintegrate. Suddenly I could no longer use the dishwasher. Showers had to be limited. Excessive toilet flushing was questioned. The wash machine had to be equipped with a long hose that could be led outside to dump water onto the bushes instead of into the septic tank.

Our driveway came into question. It was made up of dirt and gravel, very long, and came uphill from the street below to the top of our hill. It had electric, phone, and water lines buried under it, but apparently, after more than twenty-five years of faultless performance, now these were unexplainably not deep enough to be safe. My husband didn't want any trucks driving on it. He preferred that people park below and walk up. His anxiety climbed with each rainstorm; the entire driveway might just wash out, taking all of our utilities with it.

He had severe bouts of anxiety over the proximity of the back road, the condition of our roof, the nearby highway, our two pet cats, the possibility of our windows leaking, black mold, poisonous snakes, people breaking into the sheds, the rapid overgrowth of weeds in our yard presenting a fire hazard…the list went on and on.

Each new item he thought of was, for him, a case for endless, *exhaustive* discussion; with him "*proving*" to me logically" why it needed our immediate attention and *must* be dealt with. And with me trying to allay his fears and offer reassurance and support, which he in turn, doubted and was unable to accept.

Meanwhile, his antipathy to heat increased in scope. He now didn't want me using the oven, or later, even the stovetop. He begged me to *please* only use our two microwave ovens to prepare meals. And even to limit that usage. Our world had shrunk to a cold, darkened place within the six rooms of our house, and was further restricted by a myriad of do's and don'ts.

In plain language, life was hell.

This all didn't happen overnight. It took months – some of it took years to develop. I read somewhere that a person can withstand untold amounts of discomfort, even torture, if only it's being applied in very tiny increments. I think I believe this. If it weren't true, I would surely have ended up being institutionalized.

Faced with the enormity of the final picture of how we wound up living, friends started drifting away – if I couldn't do anything for him, how could they? If the combination of family, time, and medical help hadn't changed anything, what was left? People who invited us to their homes out of the kindness of their hearts – or possibly out of pity, no longer did. After one or two experiences, I'm pretty sure they cringed at the very idea of a repeat.

One of our daughters who happened to live in the nearby town, tried to get us out of the house and over to her place at least once a week. After years of effort, even she was eventually overwhelmed by the demands, the stress, and the sheer inability of *anyone* to make things right for him, no matter how hard they tried.

We never lacked for suggestions; advice poured in for the entire length of time, well intentioned and sincere. Everyone had their own pet theory, a very logical cause, and a sure-cure remedy. Try a change of scenery? He was too incapacitated by anxiety and depression to try. Perhaps a mental institution might help with intense therapy? To satisfy me, he entered a mental ward at the hospital. It lasted two days. It obviously wasn't the answer. They didn't have anything new to offer. How can you even begin to treat something when you don't know what it is?

Perhaps he needed to eat an abundance of red meat and get lots of exercise? Meat might be good, but exercise incapacitated him. Maybe he could leave home and enter a nursing home / rehab / assisted living facility? He was frightened and horrified – he didn't feel ready to give up and die. I too, was disturbed by the idea, although I have to admit, there was a part of me that yearned terribly for the relief.

Wait a minute. The relief? What had I been thinking all these months and years? How was I managing to cope with all the aspects of this – the ending of all activities? Of all fun. The abrupt stop to all socialization? No more friends? The deprivation of normal daily life? Having to struggle with minimal water use, microwave-only food, a dark, cold environment?

It sounds funny, even ridiculous, but I don't know the answer. It just happened and somehow I managed to live through it. The kids were calling me Saint Mom, but that's not it…I'm certainly not a saint. So many things that I thought were really important to me…went by the wayside. Our children were sad for me, for us both; they were heartbroken. They were angry for me, for us both. And they were outraged that their parents should be stuck in such a twisted, abnormal situation.

And on top of their sorrow, anger and frustration, I'm sure they all felt that they were being rejected. Increasingly throughout his illness, he refused phone calls, didn't want visits from anyone. As the disease progressed he was aware of his diminished ability, and felt embarrassed by it. He didn't want anyone – even his children – to see him that way. It may have felt right to him to do that, but it was not right for his children. Time and again, they felt rejected. They were deeply hurt.

I do have feelings, I really do. I'm not a saint, and I'm not some kind of stuffed dummy who just sat there and took it without any reaction on my part. I reasoned with my husband – hours of reasoning, long and hard. And I pleaded. I begged. I threatened, gave ultimatums. I raged and yelled, pushed to the brink, ready to smash windows and walls. And I often wept bitterly – with him and alone in the other room or on the phone with family members.

What did I do to occupy those hours of isolation? I read. Dozens of books. I became a crossword puzzle addict – variety puzzles. I took out my frustrations in brain games. And there were hours of television. I spent time on the phone, with friends, and then later with family. My outdoor exercise diminished and finally stopped; he did not want to be left alone. He actually became frightened of being alone.

Could I have walked out? It was suggested many times. *That* I could not do. No matter how bitter or resentful or absolutely, unfairly *imprisoned* I felt, there was still always the question of duty. Of obligation. Of being bound by marriage vows. Doesn't it say quite clearly, "in sickness and in health"? And hadn't we always held to those vows, both of us, no matter what?

We cared for each other. For our entire fifty-six years together, we were best friends; having adventures together, laughing…and he talked with me, about everything. He was truly *interested* in my opinions. We learned together, we enjoyed things together. He kept me laughing our whole life. And he loved me. I know beyond the shadow of a doubt, that if I had been the one who was afflicted, he would never leave me.

Never.

I loved him. Oh, yes. Of course I did. How else could anyone stick with such a complex, often-difficult man? So I stayed throughout his illness. And I coped. And somehow, I endured.

CHAPTER 5

After about 3 years of deteriorating conditions and increasing desperation on my part, I convinced him to move back to Wisconsin. Another daughter lived there, our oldest, who was now retired and had time enough to help me in this battle; to ferry us to medical appointments, to assist with household duties, and to try to keep me sane and healthy. By then, my health had begun to suffer – remember – I was three and a half years older than my husband was. I was seventy-eight when we moved.

I would hope there is no misunderstanding here – seven children and only one could offer help? No. Everyone did help. *However* they could. *When* they could. As *much* as they were able. Of course some, at different times, were able to do more than others were. During the first years, while we were still in Arizona, the burden of driving, shopping assistance, care giving and other endless small tasks fell to the daughter who lived close by. Although she had a large family and worked full-time, she did what she could.

Then later, in Wisconsin, one son who was living within a couple hours of driving distance would often come to spell me, to give me a precious afternoon to go shopping with our daughter. On occasion, he would stay long enough for me to have an entire weekend. But he too, had a family and a job.

Here is where life intercedes with its demands and constraints, and presents us with the hard facts of reality. Everyone had jobs. And families. And lived in distant states. Would *any* older person, even in my position of genuine need, want their children to uproot their lives, set their families aside, or put their jobs in jeopardy? I don't think so. I know that I certainly didn't.

* * *

When moving time arrived, I gave away the couch. It gave me great pleasure to do that – almost like shedding an old dirty skin that clung and suffocated. The sofa had become a symbol of what ailed him; he stopped living and took to the couch. The living room sofa had become his refuge and also my rival. He preferred it to me...

Two of our children came to Arizona to

pack up our household, sell off two travel trailers, a truck, and our home. We couldn't have done it alone. We took an apartment near our older daughter in southeast Wisconsin. A few things did change for us. My husband no longer could agonize over a questionable septic tank and a *faulty* driveway. And now I could use the dishwasher, I could shower to my heart's delight, and flush ten times if I pleased.

* * *

The apartment was still cold though. And the blinds were shut, so it remained dark. And I could still only use a microwave to cook. However, I could now leave my husband watching TV while I walked to the other end of the complex to have coffee with my daughter. If I needed her, she was available – she was retired. I had more help with shopping. And I had some company on a daily basis now. Which was wonderful, since my husband had stopped having any conversation beyond a few words with me. He most often only voiced his needs or answered my questions.

And I could again laugh with someone…Oh, my, how important that is! Maybe we don't miss it until it's gone. From the very beginning of his illness, my husband had lost his sense of humor, his appreciation and enjoyment of fun. Indeed, the very spark of life had vanished and he'd become an empty shell, serious, blank-faced, hardly even remotely resembling the lively, responsive man he had once been. If I laughed on the phone with my kids, it rang hollow in our quiet home.

It seems odd to reflect that his beginning symptoms never changed or became very numerous. Just that handful: dizziness, feeling too hot, sensitivity to light, anxiety, loss of humor. You would think that in an eight to ten year span of illness, there would be more. Some kind of change. But that didn't happen.

What are the symptoms of Lewy Body Dementia? Nothing specific. What does testing show? Nothing specific. How puzzling.

Of course that was then. *Before* we knew about Lewy Body Dementia. According to more recent research, specifically on the LBD Association website, the most common symptoms include:

- Impaired thinking, such as loss of

executive function (planning, processing information) memory, or the ability to understand visual information.

- Fluctuations in cognition, attention or alertness.

- Problems with movement including tremors, stiffness, slowness and difficulty walking

- Visual hallucinations (seeing things that are not present)

- Sleep disorders, such as acting out one's dreams while asleep.

- Behavioral and mood symptoms, including depression, apathy, anxiety, agitation, delusions or paranoia

• Changes in autonomic body functions, such as blood pressure control, temperature regulation, bladder and bowel function.

Of the above symptoms, my husband's were few. Along with the dizziness, there were some mood changes and the sudden intolerance to heat. Of course, the inevitable physical changes did start to take place. No one can lead a completely sedentary life and not look the part. Before the onset of his illness, at the age of seventy, he had appeared to be more like he was between forty and fifty. That changed; he started a steady gain in weight. He no longer stood erect; he slumped. He looked defeated. Perhaps it was no wonder that so many people thought his entire problem was just severe depression.

He gradually became weaker too. The non-use of major muscle groups eventually results in major weakness. He started using a walker, first outdoors and then later he used it around the house. It was increasingly difficult for him to get in and out of bed, in and out of cars, or even to get himself up off the couch.

In the second year of living in Wisconsin, we moved to a small town in the center of the state and took an apartment just four doors down from our daughter's. During the next four years, several more little changes appeared, and I can only guess if these might be from LBD. At the time they seemed to be due to his physical debilitation. He began to have episodes of falling down – but only at night when he was roaming the kitchen seeking his midnight snacks. I could always tell when he'd been up at night snacking by the spilled liquids and trail of half-opened packages.

There was some ongoing difficulty with urinary control; he requested a urinal be available at night for accident prevention. It was unclear if this was from a prostate problem or from an increasing physical weakness. My laundry duties increased, nonetheless. He also had recurring bouts of constipation, so that too became a daily concern involving worry and medication.

He started having some minor tremors that would mysteriously come and go. Then later he developed unusual leg cramps, mostly in his right leg. The front thigh muscle would tighten up into a painful knot several times a day. Meanwhile the doctor visits and parade of prescriptions continued. One medic absolutely ruled out Parkinson's disease. How he reached that conclusion on only one visit escapes me.

A new development before his final year was dreams and hallucinations. Our cat had died four years earlier, but he now thought she was back. He would see her on the couch, curled up, sleeping. Or on the foot of his bed. He occasionally thought he saw things crawling on the carpeting or on the walls.

His dreams became vivid. He would

awaken me at night, shouting at some unknown adversary in his sleep. Or flailing about, knocking over a lamp or bumping into the wall. Several times he fell out of bed. Sleepwalking became a problem and everyone worried about the hazards *that* presented. The family debated and agonized over what to do. Eventually the decision was taken completely out of our hands.

CHAPTER 6

On the evening of January 7, 2014, our apartment was flooded when pipes burst in the apartment upstairs from us. Our daughter immediately moved us into a motel. While there she brought us meals, clean clothing, and news of the progress being made on the apartment cleanup. My husband continued to watch TV during the day, but his nights became even more disturbed.

We had to live in the motel for a full month, and during that time he became more distant mentally – not quite in touch with reality, and his confusion was much more noticeable at night - every night. He would wake me to ask where the bathroom was or to request some food. He had confusion over where his bed was. My ongoing research informed me about the "Sundowner syndrome". Sundowning, or sundown syndrome, affects some people who have Alzheimer's disease and dementia. A person with dementia who "sundowns" can get confused and agitated as the sun goes down, and sometimes throughout the night. Sundowning may prevent people with dementia from sleeping well. It may also make them more likely to *wander*.

The turning point came one morning when I discovered a bad scrape and bruising on his arm and knee. When I asked about it, he said he thought he'd fallen- maybe. And he related a "dream" about going out into the hallway to "look for something" and not being able to find his way back to our room again.

It wasn't a dream, of course, for I found the door unlocked and partly ajar, and out in the hallway on the wall was a scrape where his walker had hit, and a bloody smear where he had fallen and shredded his elbow. While I was worrying about all this, he turned from the TV and asked if I could locate a urinal or something – he didn't think he could make it to the bathroom anymore; he couldn't walk at all.

* * *

An ambulance took him to the hospital, and two or three days later, to a nursing home. He hated it. There they tried physical therapy, occupational therapy, and tried to interest him in some gentle socialization. They had no more luck in the year he lived there, than I'd had in all of the previous years. He was verbal enough to complain some, he was very pleasant to all the staff, but he only wanted to keep to himself in his room, sit in the recliner and watch TV.

Several months later he started exhibiting paranoid ideas. He had his mustache and beard shaved off; convinced they would cause the staff to be prejudiced against him. He suspected the room was bugged; the ceiling sprinkler system had microphones. The nurses down the hall were talking about him. He allowed no family pictures in his room because "they" would know who his family was and bad things would happen. And he allowed no decorations; his excuse – someone might steal them.

His private room at the nursing home remained dark and cold; he had me purchase a window AC unit. While everyone else's rooms were warm, inviting, cozy places decorated with items from home such as lamps, pictures of family, comfortable furnishings – his room stayed empty and institutional and impersonal.

During the last several months, both he and the staff people told me of his continuing and increasing hallucinations. He saw multiple cats now. He was convinced some of them slept with him. He worried a bit over whether they were being taken care of and fed properly, but he didn't really mind their presence. He occasionally thought one or another family member was there, or heard their voices out in the hallway.

He refused phone calls from family, again causing them rejection and heartache. He told me he just didn't know what to talk about. Carrying on a conversation had become too difficult. He balked at the idea of having visitors. We tried to force a few, but that agitated him severely. One daughter tried several times, bringing him ice cream and a small device for listening to his favorite music, and suggested watching movies with him. He would nod and agree that maybe he could, but it was really beyond his ability; when we were alone he would say, "I can't." A phrase he used incessantly. "I can't." A phrase I'd come to loathe. He sometimes tried to put forth an effort, but he truly couldn't sustain it.

Early on, the people at the nursing home told me that he occasionally joked with them. I never saw it. They said he always remembered everyone's name. This I can believe – he had a phenomenal memory. I got the feeling that he talked more with them all during that last year than he did with me. He wanted *me* to visit as *often* as I could and stay as long as possible, but while I was there, he most often spent the time dozing or just resting with his eyes closed. In the first several months, I visited him every day. Gradually my visits decreased to 6 times a week, then to 5, and finally to 3. Towards the end, he barely knew I was there.

He began doing imaginary things with his hands held out in front of him – as though he were turning a screwdriver or fixing an intricate, detailed object, or tightening a bottle top. He would pick up invisible small things from the table or from his lap and carefully put them into his shirt pocket. All with his eyes closed tight. At times, he handed them to me to dispose of.

The abbreviated conversations that we did have were almost always about the children, especially in the beginning. He would ask about each of them, nod at my answers, and try to extend the conversation, but it was apparent that although he was interested in what was taking place in their lives, it was too difficult for him to concentrate; his eyes would drift to the TV, or in later months, droop and close. More than once he tried to explain that he just couldn't think anymore, and sometimes when he would make an attempt to tell me something, he'd say, "it's just too complicated," and he didn't know what to say next.

For a long time, he cut down on food,

claiming loss of appetite or dislike of food options. The truth of the matter was that his paranoia now included the phrase, "They're trying to poison me." He dropped to 113 pounds and shrunk drastically in height. The last two or three months, he stopped watching TV completely.

Eventually he agreed to hospice care, and I believe that was a good thing. Those people are wonderfully kind and compassionate. They really do care. They worked diligently to make him more comfortable, massaged his arms and legs with lotion, and visited him when I couldn't be there. There were many other small kindnesses.

It wasn't until the last month that his family doctor – who continued to see him at the nursing home – mentioned Lewy Body Dementia as a possible diagnosis. He also mentioned Shy Drager and Parkinson's symptoms, so he still wasn't really certain. And how could he be? I've been told that only autopsy gives definitive answers. Examining the brain cells. I found too, that LBD is second only to Alzheimer's in frequency of occurrence. That surprised me. Everyone knows Alzheimer's; no one knows

LBD.

Another piece of information I turned up said that Lewy Body Dementia shows itself in the very early stages with radical change in sleep patterns and disruptive dreams that are violent, vivid and frightening. And I recalled that, as early as two years previous to my husband becoming dizzy, he *had* started having those types of dreams. In his sleep, he would physically fight with people, thrashing around wildly, lashing out. Or he'd be chased by some large, deadly animal and have to struggle violently to escape. And he would walk in his sleep, going from room to room, waking up badly disoriented, standing in the kitchen in front of an open refrigerator. Or, perversely, he'd have weeks-long bouts of insomnia. These were the same symptoms that recurred during his last year or two.

In retrospect, what answer would we have preferred? The years-long mystery we had? Or some label? And what label would we want applied? Lewy Body Syndrome. Lewy Body Disease. Lewy Body Dementia. And it's that last one that scares the pants off everyone. "Syndrome" sounds almost benign and non-threatening as a "quirk" an "idiosyncrasy". And "disease" seems to be something you might catch, like a cold or the flu - or even develop from some deficiency of a vitamin, or from a betrayal of blood cells or a malfunctioning organ.

Oh, but that word "dementia". That word makes strong men run and hide. The word "dementia" says raving maniac, doesn't it? Or sitting in the corner, drooling, regarding the floor with a vacant stare? Or some unfortunate, twisted existence that oscillates between those extremes? We all think this. And we all fear this.

Not only does the word "dementia"

isolate a person socially, it calls into the question *all* of their past actions, their habits, their decisions. It gives people – not all, but some people – permission to squint judiciously and say, "You know, I always *thought* there was something really strange about him…"

* * *

My husband's last two or three weeks were indicative of how LBD ends. No outcry, no shock, no fear. In his case, at any rate, it was a gradual, very slow withdrawal of awareness. Almost a gentle falling asleep. It was obvious that he wasn't suffering; he was finally at peace. In his last moments, he raised his arms just a little, let them drop, and then he was gone.

* * *

All of his cares are over now. Our family has gathered from their distant places for our particular kind of memorial. We have talked into the wee hours, eaten together; we have, as always, tossed opinions at each other, we have laughed a lot, until our sides hurt. And of course we have all done our crying. My husband, their father, was much in our minds and in our hearts and he will surely remain there. We all have many memories, good and bad, old and new.

He is well remembered.

AFTERWORD

My hope in writing this is, first and foremost, that it helps to give some measure of peace to my children. Either in answering any questions they might have or to give them a better understanding of LBD. Not the science of it. They are all intelligent; they've looked it up. But an understanding of the personal side of it, and the small details. And perhaps a better insight into my thoughts and feelings, the inner workings of my struggle in playing out the role of main caregiver. I know in their hearts, they fought right alongside of me, each of them, every step of the way.

And then too, if there is any small bit of information, or shred of support or even just a feeling of kinship that other caregivers can derive from these pages – that would make me happy. If any person who is dealing with some sort of mental deterioration in a loved one, would seek any advice from me, I would suggest this: look for support groups. In retrospect, I wish I had done so.

A good place to start might be at the Lewy Body Dementia Association website, right here:

http://www.lbda.org/category/3437/what-is-lbd.htm

Meanwhile, the research is ongoing and more is understood with every passing day in the field of brain cell diseases. Perhaps the future may hold alleviation of symptoms or even a cure.

I certainly hope so.

ABOUT THE AUTHOR

Barbara J. Secklin is 84 years young. She has seven children who include retired business owners, published authors, a college professor, a physicist, teachers, and a computer tech. She also has 19 grandchildren, and 15 great-grandchildren. After a 30-plus year love affair with the state of Arizona, she moved back to her home state of Wisconsin, but still cannot get used to the winters. Besides writing poetry, she's enjoyed many creative pursuits through the years, some of which are painting, pottery and sculpture, designing jewelry, and teaching wire wrapping and weaving. While in Arizona she also spent time camping, hiking, and swimming; and together with her husband of nearly 56 years, traveling the United States - exploring many of the National Parks.

Barbara is an avid reader and puzzle-book aficionado, which in turn, some claim, has turned her into a walking thesaurus. She now spends most mornings as the editor of her daughter's novels, for which she is paid exorbitant amounts of coffee. In the future, she plans to co-author a novel with said daughter, and one day hopes to revisit her beloved Arizona.

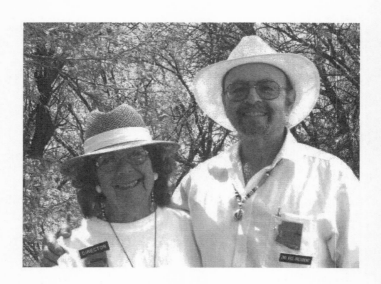

Printed in Great Britain
by Amazon.co.uk, Ltd.,
Marston Gate.